CIRCULATING WITH THE LISTED PROBLEM(S):

Pencil marks throughout
4-30-10 mm

√

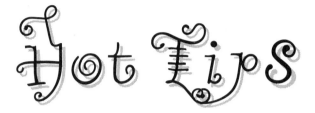

Hot Tips

Step-by-Step Nail Art
You Can Create at Home!

Sandra Marion

Photographs by Colette Monción

Crown Trade Paperbacks
New York

Copyright © 1996 by Crown Publishers, Inc.

Published by Crown Trade Paperbacks, 201 East 50th Street, New York, New York 10022. Member of the Crown Publishing Group.

Random House, Inc. New York, Toronto, London, Sydney, Auckland

http://www.randomhouse.com/

CROWN TRADE PAPERBACKS and colophon are trademarks of Crown Publishers, Inc.

Printed in the United States of America.

Library of Congress Cataloging-in-Publication Data is available upon request.

ISBN 0-517-88614-6

10 9 8 7 6 5 4 3 2 1

First Edition

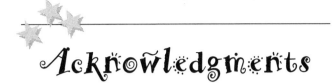

Acknowledgments

This book could not have come to pass without the gracious help of the professionals at the salons at which nail fashion trends are created:

Jatae Hair Studio
New York, New York

Casablanca Nail Salon
New York, New York

Q-1 Nails
New York, New York

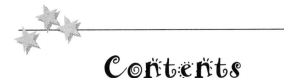

Contents

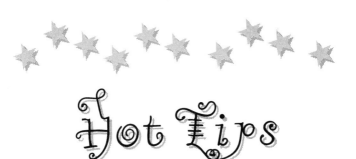

Hot Tips

introduction

They can cook spaghetti or type a letter, lace up your running shoes or turn the pages of a book. For all their functionality, the hands are also incredibly expressive. They can even go the face one better, by entering the realm of art—and this is what *Hot Tips* is all about.

This book will help you see your nails as ten tiny canvases, on which you'll create unique designs using airbrush and appliqués, glitter and color, and the latest nail design techniques and tools. You'll also learn more about nail care and how to keep your hands looking their best.

Create bright designs for your next birthday bash, or a patriotic theme for the Fourth of July. Here are ideas for Halloween, Thanksgiving, or Christmas, plus far-out designs for nights at the club, or for whenever you just feel like expressing yourself. Bring your friends in on the action, and make a few bucks preparing their nails for the next big event!

Using the techniques here, there's no limit to your creativity. Take advantage of *Hot Tips*, and enjoy!

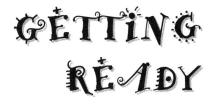

GETTING READY

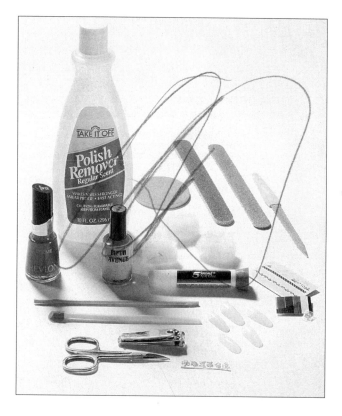

Tools of the Trade

These are the essential tools you'll need for manicuring your nails and maintaining their health. All items are readily available at drugstores or beauty salons. Some even come in kits.

Base Coat

The base coat is applied before polish. It acts as an adhesive, preventing polish from peeling away, and also protects the nail from absorbing any dyes that are in the polish.

Buffers

Buffers, as the name implies, help give a finishing shine to your nail. Most come with multiple surfaces for the different steps involved in buffing your nails.

Cuticle Clippers

Optional. They're good for trimming the cuticle or removing hangnails—but cuticle trimming is usually unnecessary, and hangnails can just as easily be cut with nail clippers.

Cuticle Cream and Cuticle Oil

These substances soften and nourish the cuticles to keep them from drying out and splitting.

Decorations

Glitter, frosted polishes, appliqués, the airbrush, stencils, foil nuggets, and other elements of decoration can be picked up in any beauty supply store.

Glue and Activator Spray

When fitting artificial nails and fiberglass nail wraps, resins and activator sprays are essential. Glue is used to bond artificial nails to your nail. Activator spray is used to create a smooth surface, eliminate streaks, and keep polish from running.

Nail Clippers

A basic tool, available everywhere. Any sharp pair will do. Smaller ones are easier to use.

Nail File

The term file generally brings to mind the metal variety—but emery boards are best. Typically finer than metal, they're gentler on the nails. Metal files (and coarser emery boards) tend to remove more of the nail with each stroke, and make subtle file work difficult.

Nail Polish

Polishes, of course, provide color, and are best used with a base coat and a top coat. Polishes are available in a wide variety of colors and glosses. Some contain glitter for added sparkle.

Nail Polish Remover

These contain organic solvents for stripping polish from nails. Polish remover without acetone is recommended for removing polish from natural as well as artificial nails. Too frequent use of removers can be drying.

Nail Strengthener

Nail strengtheners harden and give support to the nail, preventing splits and tears. Nail strengthener is applied under the base coat.

Orange Sticks

Useful for pushing back the cuticle. Rubber tipped ends are gentler. If your orange stick lacks a rubber tip, wrap the tip in a bit of cotton to make it softer.

Top Coat

Applied over dry polish, appliqués, and other elements, the top coat is a tough sealant which adds gloss to the nail.

The Manicure

Manicuring done by yourself or by a friend gets the nails in good condition before decorations are applied. Using good technique to bring your nails to their peak condition is easy, therapeutic, and relaxing.

Be sure to remove old polish completely before starting the manicure. For each nail, first use a fresh cotton ball moistened with non-acetone nail polish remover to soak and loosen the polish. Wait until the polish dissolves before wiping the nail clean, and you make less of a mess.

The typical manicure involves these main steps: cuticle care, trimming, filing, and buffing.

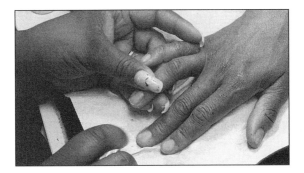

Therapy for Your Cuticles

No matter what condition your nails are in, they won't look their best next to dried, splitting, or frayed cuticles. The cuticle is the ridge of flesh at the base of the nail. Maintenance of the cuticle involves moisturizing it and pushing it back to achieve an oval shape on the nail's surface.

You'll need cuticle cream and warm soapy water to moisturize the cuticles, an orange stick to push them back, and cuticle or nail clippers to trim them. Clean up requires a soft towel.

Manicure Step 1

- Dip into the cuticle cream with your orange stick, and dab a bit onto your cuticle. Massage it in well with your thumb. Repeat for each finger. You may also brush on cuticle oil. The massage will soften your cuticles and increase blood flow to them.

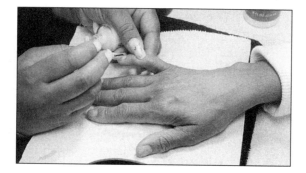

- Soak the fingertips in soapy warm water for two minutes. Be sure the water is not too hot—wrinkled fingers and cuticles can obscure the end result of your manicure. Dry thoroughly before moving on to the next step.

- Now that the cuticles are pliable, use the orange stick to gently push them back. If you find the orange stick feels too hard, use one with a rubber end, or wrap the end of your orange stick with a bit of cotton. If you experience pain when pushing your cuticles back, you're pushing too hard. Soften them further and try again.

- The best time to get rid of those hangnails is while they're soft. If you choose to remove excess cuticle, take care not to overcut. Use the cuticle clippers or nail cutters to carefully trim any hangnails from around each of your nails. Trimming the cuticle is usually unnecessary, and some manicurists say that trimming it too often only makes it grow back thicker.

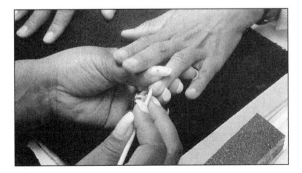

Trimming the Nail

How short should you trim your nails? That depends on your lifestyle. While long nails are sexy and glamorous, no one who types, cooks, or is active in sports can keep very long nails. The good news is that moderately short nails can look just as good as long nails when they're cared for properly.

A good gauge of how long you should keep your nails is your preoccupation with them. If you find that you're spending a lot of time taking care of your nails, they're too long for your lifestyle. If you can keep them looking good and forget about them most of the time, they're just right.

Generally, filing the nail to maintain its shape and perfect length is recommended over clipping it. Of course, taking length off the nail with a file is not always practical. That's when a nail clipper comes in handy.

Some manicurists maintain that nail clippers are more prone to split the nail, and recommend that home manicurists use scissors when taking length off the nail. Another school of thought, however, holds that the use of dull scissors is an invitation for disaster. Dull instruments of either type lead to bad results. Sharp clippers are about as good as sharp scissors, so use whichever you're more accustomed to.

There's one case, however, in which you should always use scissors, and that's if you're aiming for a square, rather than a rounded, shape. Clippers are designed to give a round shape to the nail edge.

Manicure Step 2

- Shaping the nail is a matter of preference. Choose a shape that will work with your planned nail design.

- If you're aiming for a square rather than a rounded shape, use scissors to make a single cut across the nail at the length you prefer.

- Round-edged nails can be achieved by using clippers to make a cut on each side of the nail, then trimming the center. If the tips look crude and angular, don't worry—the final shape will be achieved with a file.

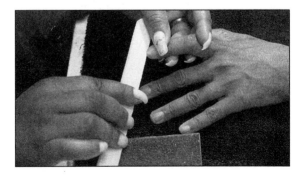

Filing the Nails

Now that you've trimmed the nails to their optimal length and approximate shape, filing is a finishing touch. To avoid splitting the nail, never use the file in a back-and-forth sawing motion or against the layers of the nail. Also avoid filing too near the cuticle at the corners of the nails. This can cause ingrown nails, and even infections.

Manicure Step 3

- File from the sides to the center of the nail, with the more abrasive side of an emery board, and then with the smoother side for light work. File in one direction only. File away from the cuticle, toward the fingertip.

- For square nails, file directly across the flat edge of the nail, in one direction only.

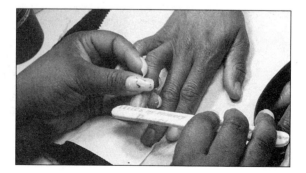

Buffing the Nail

A final step before applying nail strengthener, any kind of decoration, or a base coat, is to buff your nails. Buffing is an important part of keeping nails healthy and shiny-looking.

The buffer smooths the nail surface and stimulates circulation in the fingertips. Use all the sections of the buffer in this process, and be sure to protect the corners of your nails from the dust that will come off of them.

Manicure Step 4

- Be sure to start with the roughest surface of the buffer and work your way to the smoothest surface.

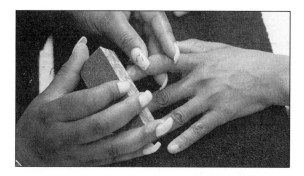

- Use baby oil and a cotton swab to collect dust from around the cuticle area. Be sure to get all the dust before applying polish—a drop or two of nail polish remover may help.

- Wipe nails clean with a cotton ball.

Your manicure is complete. Now you have two options. Take a look at your nails. If they're terrific, go directly to the second section of this book to learn how to apply exciting nail decorations to them. If they seem too short, too small, or too irregularly shaped to hold a design well, read the next page to learn about artificial nails, a perfect canvas for Hot Tips.

Artificial intelligence

A rtificial nails have come a long way from the crude, thick monstrosities adorning the fingers of yesteryear's socialites. Today's artificial nails provide a convincing alternative to natural nails, which may take years to grow to perfect length and shape. They can add glamour to your hands in an instant, or repair the one broken nail that's ruining your otherwise perfect set. They also allow your natural nails to grow underneath, protected. And they come right off with artificial nail remover. Nail polish remover with acetone can also remove artificial nails.

Use artificial nails to show off your more elaborate creations, and if you take care when removing them, you can wear them again. You can buy them at any beauty supply store. They come in quantities of 25, 100, or 200. Choose between two styles: regular or curved. You'll also need special glue to attach the nails, as well as activator spray to smooth the surface of the nail, and lotion to massage the fingers.

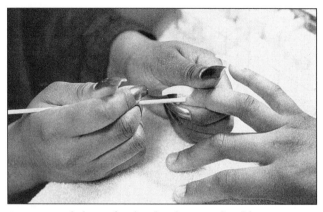

Step 1•Match the artificial nail to the natural nail from corner to corner.

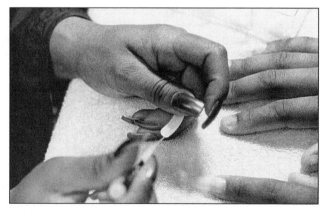

Step 2• Apply glue to the underside of the artificial nail and place over the natural nail.

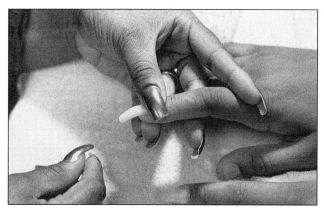

Step 3 • Press the nail in place until it holds.

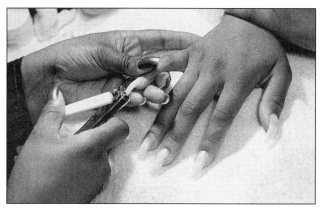

Step 4 • Trim the artificial nail with clippers.

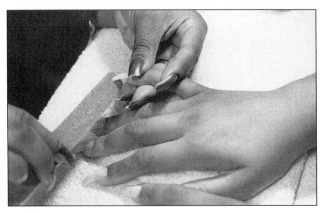

Step 5 • File and buff.

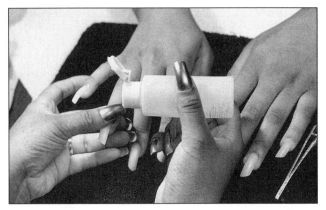

Step 6 • Coat the surface of the nail with activator. Buff and shine.

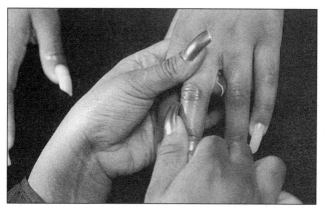

Step 7 • Massage fingers to increase circulation. Now you're ready to create some artwork!

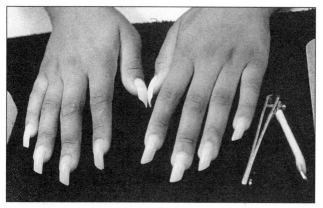

A complete set of nails filed at an angle.

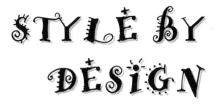

STYLE BY DESIGN

Beautifying Your Nails

Polish

Clear is clean and natural, yet elegant. Red is sultry, seductive, formal. Black is vampirish, punk, playful. Applying color or shine to your nails is a fun, easy way to accentuate any outfit or occasion.

Of course, we all know how to paint our nails, don't we? Surely there's no right or wrong way to do it? Well, that depends on whether you're aiming to just paint your nails, or if you want to paint them so they look *great*.

For stunning nails, you'll need a base polish, a colored polish, a clear top coat to harden and protect the nail, and a quick-dry polish. Now follow these rules of thumb:

- Always apply a base coat. The base coat will help polish adhere to your nails, preventing chips and cracks, and will keep your nails free of the dyes that are in the polish. You may also want to apply nail strengthener before the base coat if you have fragile or brittle nails.

- Try to leave a slight space between the polish and your cuticles. It looks better, and you won't have to apply polish remover to your cuticles when changing or taking off the polish. Polish remover can dry the cuticles.

- For rich, strong color, apply two coats of polish.

    1. Apply first coat sparingly, in three strokes: one at the center of the nail, one at the outer edge, one at the other edge. A light first coat should dry within minutes.

    2. Apply a heavier coat in the same three-stroke manner. If polish runs too thick from the brush, keep an orange stick handy for dabbing up the excess.

- A clear top coat finishes the job.

- Allow half an hour for nails to dry. Nails feel dry long before that, but the polish may still smudge.

Applying Nail Decorations

Now you're ready to go. First we'll show you how to decorate your nails with exciting adhesive stripes, decals, glitter, and gems. Then we'll show you a variety of different designs you can create freehand using a thin brush and a variety of colored polishes (check a drugstore or beauty supply store for kits).

Follow these basic steps when applying decorations to your manicured nails:

- Select your design.
- Apply two base coats and two coats of color.
- Allow nails to dry completely.
- Apply element or painted image.
- Allow nails to dry.
- Seal with top coat.

Adhesive Stripes

Adhesive stripes are made of colored foil that can be cut to form lines and shapes. Using tweezers or cuticle clippers, peel off a length of adhesive stripe from its backing. Apply to the nail, and trim using cuticle clippers. Lay the stripe across the nail, taking care to work from points nearest the cuticle to points nearest the tip of the nail.

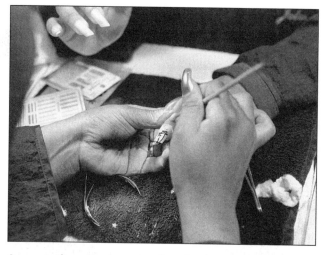

Separate the adhesive stripe from backing and slide it onto nail.

Decals

Decals are small, cut-out designs applied to the nails. Leaves, objects, flowers, and geometrics are all available in kits found in most drugstores. Decals are applied by separating them from their paper backing (a small amount of water may be necessary). Slide the decal onto the polished nail surface. Be sure to let the nail and decal dry thoroughly before applying top coat.

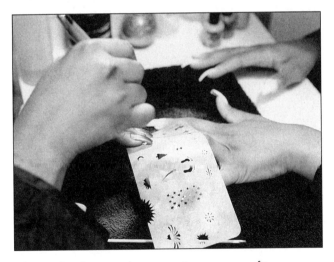

Choose decals to match an occasion or your outfit.

Glitter Polish

Glitter polish is nail polish mixed with glitter particles to add sparkle to your nails. It is applied in the same manner as regular polish, and you can often buy it packaged in convenient kits.

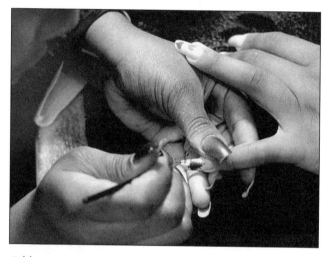

Add one or more coats of glitter polish to the manicured nail. Let nail dry between each coat.

Small Elements

Small plastic elements, like diamonds and pebbles, can be picked up with the moistened end of an orange stick and placed onto the tacky surface of a polished nail. Secure these elements by pressing them gently into the polish. The top coat will seal them in place. You can use diamonds to add brilliant accents to your nail design. You can use pebbles to add dimension and texture.

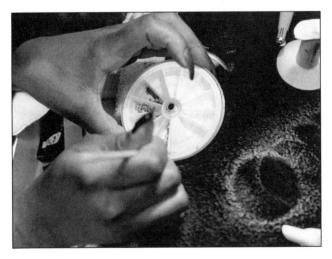

Apply small elements like diamonds, glitter, and pebbles to polished nail before it dries.

Freehand Designs

Your manicured and beautifully polished nails are ready for decoration. You may accent your hands by designing one or all of your nails. Repeat the same design or tell a story using your nails as the pages. With a paintbrush and a little imagination, your nail art can match the events in your life or mark those special days of the calendar. Here are some sample designs you can use to celebrate the season, a new romance, or any holiday.

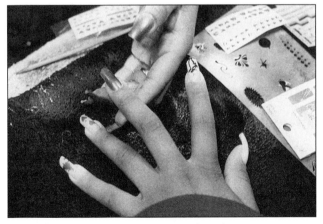

You can put a different design on each nail.

Florals

You know what they say about April showers! Welcome springtime in style with these easy-to-create freehand floral patterns. Just use color on top of a base coat, giving each part of the design enough time to dry so that the colors don't blend.

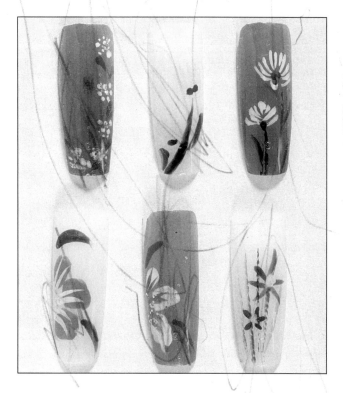

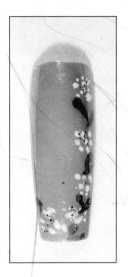

Climbing vine

Apply two coats of red polish. Allow to dry thoroughly. Paint stem of flower. Allow to dry. Paint yellow blossoms. Allow to dry. Paint green leaves. Allow to dry. Seal with top coat.

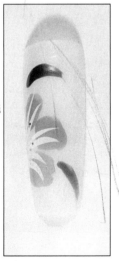

Petals

Paint the nail surface with two coats of pale pink polish. Allow to dry thoroughly. Paint three red petals with three strokes of the nail polish brush. Let dry thoroughly. Using the pale polish, paint two thin lines in each petal. Before the paint dries completely, sprinkle a few tiny bits of glitter on the pale lines. Let dry. Add green leaves as accents. Let dry. Seal with top coat.

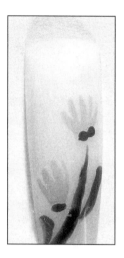

Yellow Blossoms

Apply two coats of ivory-colored polish. Let dry thoroughly between coats. Paint two large flower blossoms with yellow polish. Let dry. With green polish, paint stems and leaves. Let dry. Seal with top coat.

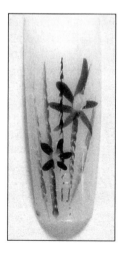

Bouquet

Apply two coats of pink polish. Allow to dry thoroughly. Use a thin brush to paint five green stems. Let dry. Paint flower blossoms purple, a short stroke for each petal. Allow to dry. Paint the center of each blossom yellow. Let dry. Seal with top coat.

Animals

Cuddly as a panda, cute as a bug, or aggressive as a tiger on the prowl. Express yourself with stylish and simple animal patterns that show the world your wild side!

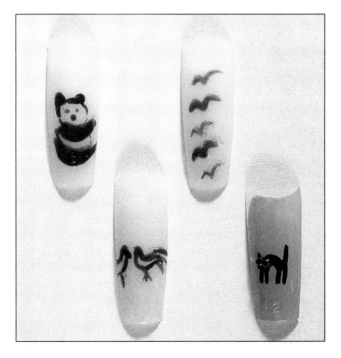

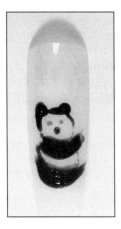

Panda

Apply two coats of off-white polish. Let the polish dry thoroughly between coats. Paint the panda on the surface of your nail using a fine brush and black polish. Practice by drawing the outline of a snowman as your base. Let dry thoroughly. Seal with top coat.

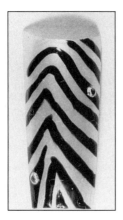

Zebra

Paint the nail surface with two coats of silver polish. Let dry. Use black nail polish to make zebra stripes. Place the diamonds before the polish dries. Let the nail dry. Seal with top coat.

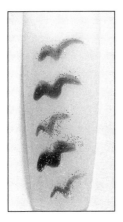

Birds in Flight

Apply two coats of ivory polish. Allow to dry thoroughly. Use gold glitter polish to paint a flock of birds. Let dry. Seal with top coat.

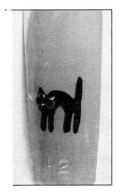

Green-eyed Black Cat

Choose two green stones and set aside. Apply two coats of orange polish. Allow to dry thoroughly. Use black polish to paint the cat. Before the cat is thoroughly dry, set two green stones for its eyes, using tweezers to pick up the stones. Let dry. Seal with top coat.

Brush Strokes

Hot Tips can be sizzling or serene. Suggest the spirit of nature with these designs.

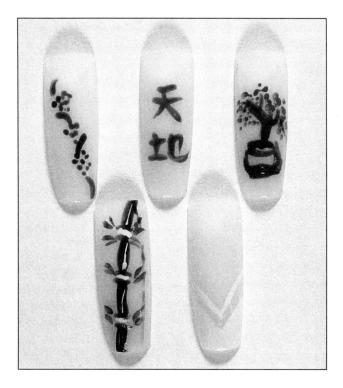

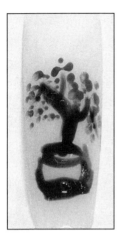

Bonsai Tree

Cut bonsai tree from a card of decals. Set aside. Apply two coats of ivory polish. Let dry thoroughly. Dip the decal in water for a second to loosen it. Slide onto nail. Blot very gently. Let dry. Seal with top coat.

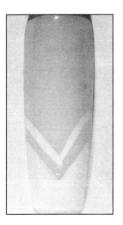

Mountain Snow

Apply two coats of ivory polish. Allow to dry completely. Paint the tip of the nail in a wide V-shaped design using white polish. Paint a thin ivory V-shaped line parallel to the one at the tip, leaving a small ivory V between the two white ones. Adhesive stripes may also be used to create the V (see p. 38 for more information on using adhesive stripes). Let dry. Seal with top coat.

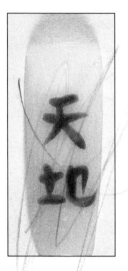

Calligraphy

Apply two coats of ivory polish. Let dry. Paint characters with thin brush and black polish. Let dry. Seal with top coat.

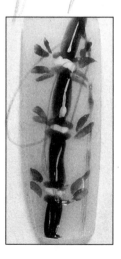

Bamboo

Apply two coats of ivory polish. Let dry. Using black polish, paint the segments of the bamboo with a slanted broken line. Let dry. Paint horizontal white lines between each segment. Paint a pencil-thin white line down the vertical center of the bamboo stalk. Let dry. Add green leaves. Let dry. Seal with top coat.

Seasonals

You'll have them saluting on the Fourth, caroling on Christmas, or howling on Halloween with these spirit-raising holiday and seasonal designs. Be the life of the party for the upcoming holiday!

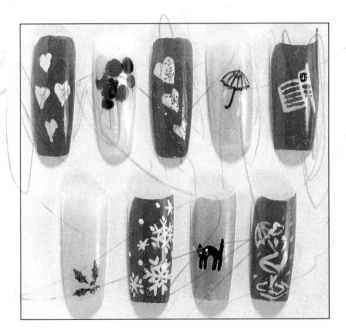

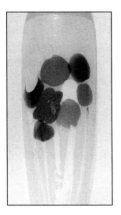

Balloons

Apply two coats of ivory nail polish. Allow to dry completely. Paint balloons by dabbing brush strokes of different colors close together. Let dry completely. Paint a few more balloons, having some overlap the first ones. Let dry completely. Paint streamers in a contrasting color. Let dry. Seal with top coat.

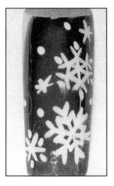

Snowflakes

Cut snowflakes from a card of decals. Set aside. Paint nails with two coats of red polish. Let dry completely. Dip the decals in water for a second to loosen them. Slide decals onto the nail. Blot gently. Let dry. Seal with top coat.

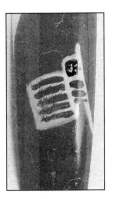

Old Glory

Apply two coats of red polish. Let dry thoroughly between coats. Paint outline and stripes of flag with white polish. Let dry. Paint the top corner of flag with blue polish. Let dry. Spot the blue with white paint for stars. Let dry. Seal with top coat.

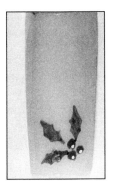

Holly or Mistletoe

Paint nails with two coats of pink polish. Allow to dry completely. Paint three leaves of holly with green polish. Let dry. With red polish, paint three berries. Let dry. Dot the berries with white polish. Let dry. Seal the nail with top coat.

Making the Scene

Use these slick party designs to become the center of attention. Let'em know who you are or who you're thinking about by putting your name or the name of someone special right on your nails. You can express your emotions with any number of fanciful faces.

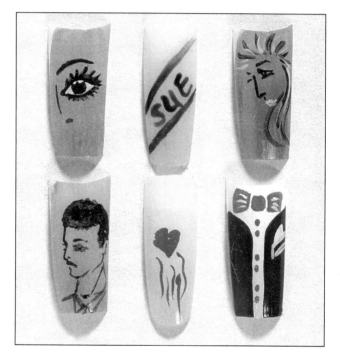

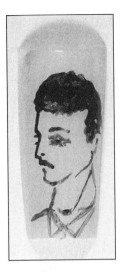

Dreamboat

Apply two coats of pink polish. Draw the head and shirt collar of a man using black polish and a thin paint brush. Let dry. Seal with top coat.

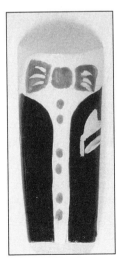

Tuxedo

Apply two coats of white polish. Allow to dry completely. Paint a stroke of black polish on each side of the nail, being sure to leave the center and tip white. Let dry. Paint buttons using red polish. Let dry. Paint red bow tie in three strokes. Brush a few lines of white paint for the pocket and handkerchief. Let dry. Seal with top coat.

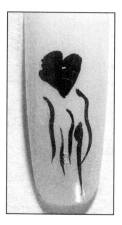

Heart's Afire

Apply two coats of ivory polish. Let dry. Paint a heart shape using two intersecting brushstrokes of red polish. Let dry. Paint flames in red or orange. Let dry. Seal with top coat.

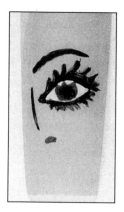

Wink

Apply two coats of pink polish. Allow to dry. Paint the white of the eye. Let dry. Paint the iris of the eye brown, blue, or green. Let dry. Paint the pupil black. Using black polish and a thin brush, draw the outline of the eye and the eyelashes. Let dry. Paint the eyebrow, a vertical line for the nose, and a short horizontal line for the mouth black. Let dry. Seal with top coat.

Landscapes

Evoke the peace and quiet of wide open spaces or the hustle and bustle of city life with these artful landscape designs. Let people know where you're from—or where you want to be!

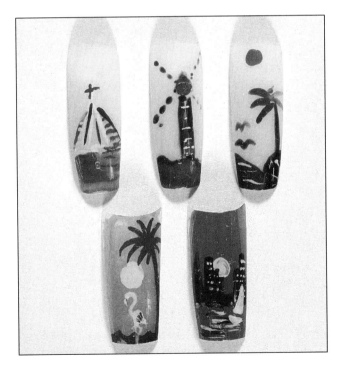

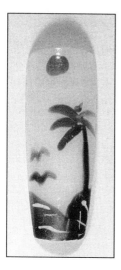

Palm Tree

Apply two coats of very pale nail polish to the surface of the nail. Allow to dry. Paint the lower left hand corner of nail sea blue. Let dry. Paint the lower right hand corner black, extending the black paint a bit over the blue sea. Let dry. Paint the trunk of the palm tree black. Let dry. Paint the palm fronds green. Let dry. Use gold glitter paint to make the birds. Let dry. Paint the sun orange. Let dry. With thin brush and white paint, draw waves in the sea. Let dry. Seal with top coat.

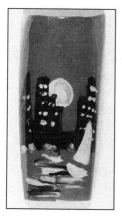

Skyline

Apply two coats of red nail polish. Allow to dry. Using black polish, paint thin brush strokes to form the buildings. Let dry. With a thin brush, dab white polish on the buildings to make windows. Let dry. Paint in a yellow sun. Paint a white sailboat or use a decal. Let dry. Make horizontal white lines near the base of the sailboat to indicate water. Let dry. Seal nail with top coat.

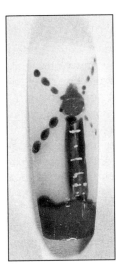

Lighthouse

Apply two coats of ivory polish. Let dry. Paint the base of the nail blue like the sea. Let dry. Use one stroke of black polish to form the lighthouse. Let dry. Paint a red circle atop the lighthouse, for the light. Let dry. Paint a small black tower above the red circle. Paint black dots radiating from the circle to indicate beams of light. Let dry. Seal with top coat.

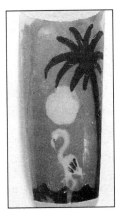

Flamingo Sun

Cut flamingo from card of decals. Set aside. Apply two coats of rose polish. Allow to dry. With black polish, paint a wavy black line at the base of the nail. Paint the trunk of the palm tree black. Let dry. Paint the palm fronds green. Let dry. Dip the flamingo decal in water for a second to loosen it. Slide onto nail. Blot very gently. Let dry. Paint a bright yellow sun. Let dry. Seal with top coat.

Abstract

High times call for high fashion. And what's high fashion without Hot Tips? Use stripes, shapes, appliqués, and freehand color to match that special outfit. What do you see in these abstract designs? And what do you see yourself wearing with them?

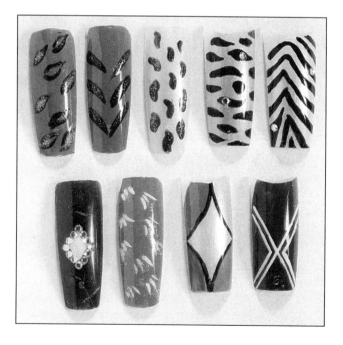

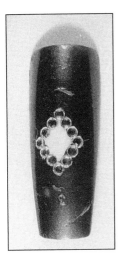

Royal Sparkle

Apply two coats of royal blue polish. Let dry. Apply two coats of white polish in the middle of your nail to form a diamond with quarter-inch sides. When the polish is slightly dry, you can set in the stones. Put a tiny bit of glue on the gems. Use tweezers to place them around the central diamond. Seal nail with top coat.

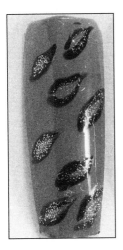

Floating Objects

Apply two coats of red polish. Let dry. Put a few dabs of gold glitter polish on the nail, being careful not to place them too far apart. Let dry. Outline each dab with black polish. Let dry. Add additional dabs, spacing as desired. Seal with top coat.

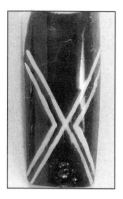

Crossroads

Cut white adhesive stripes from card and set aside. Apply two coats of burgundy polish. Let dry. To make the X, lift one adhesive stripe and place it on the nail at a diagonal. Cross the second stripe over it. Using white polish, paint V-shaped lines on the right and left sides of the adhesive-stripe X. Seal with top coat.

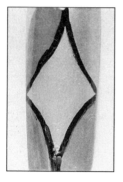

Diamond

Paint a gold diamond shape in the center of the nail. Let dry. Outline the diamond with black polish. Let dry. Paint each corner of the nail a different color, like red, purple, orange, and green. Let dry. Seal with top coat.

Fixing Tips

Repairing Polish

Even with the proper application of base coat and polish, it's possible that your polish may chip or smudge. Sometimes you can repair a chip by buffing over the damaged area. Use a lightweight buffer to avoid removing more polish than necessary. Then apply a light layer of polish over the affected area. Finally, when the nail is dry to the touch, it's safe to paint a top coat over the entire nail.

You can repair a smudge in a similar way. Just moisten polish with a drop of base coat. Polish over it with color and top coat.

Removing Stray Polish and Glue

If the polish or glue that you're working with spills over onto your finger, remove it with nail polish remover. If you're painting fine details and make a mistake, you can fix it with the tip of an orange stick covered with cotton.

And Remember . . .

If you really don't like the way your design turned out, you can always remove it and start again. Or use dark polish to paint over the mistake, and start from scratch with a new design!

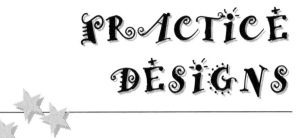

PRACTICE DESIGNS

Practice Tips

ere are some practice templates. You can use these to draw your designs first, before painting them. Experiment and have fun!

Draw your design here

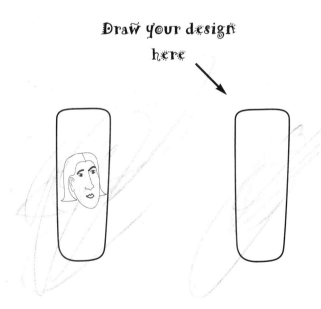

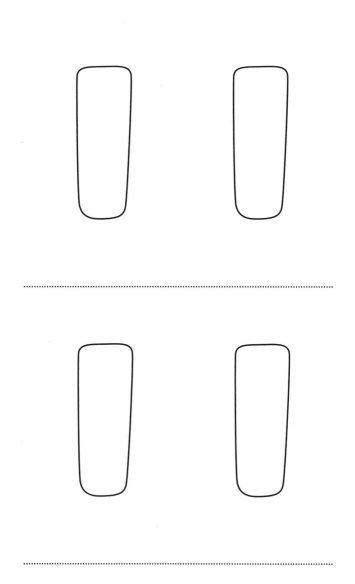

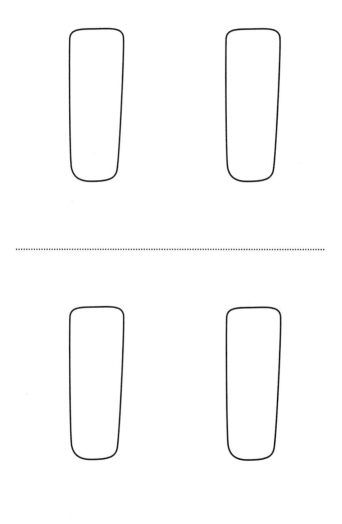

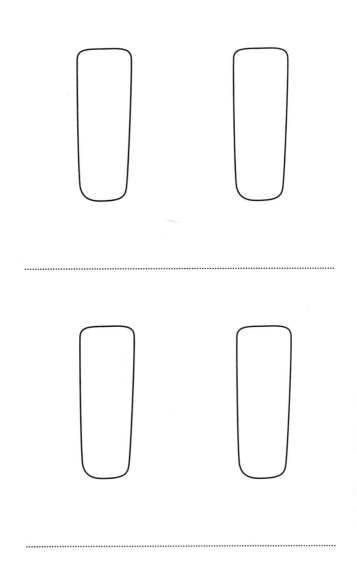

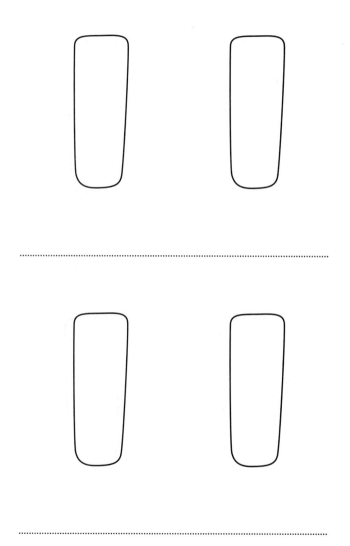

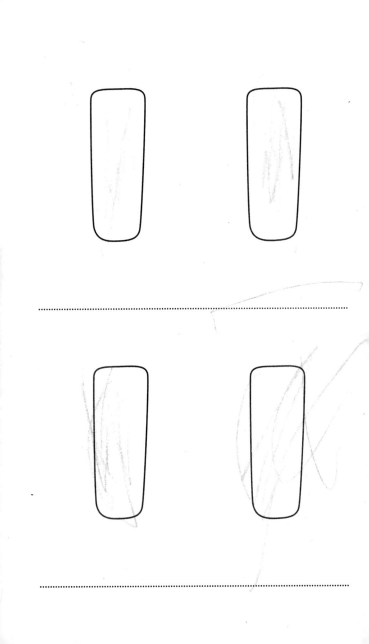

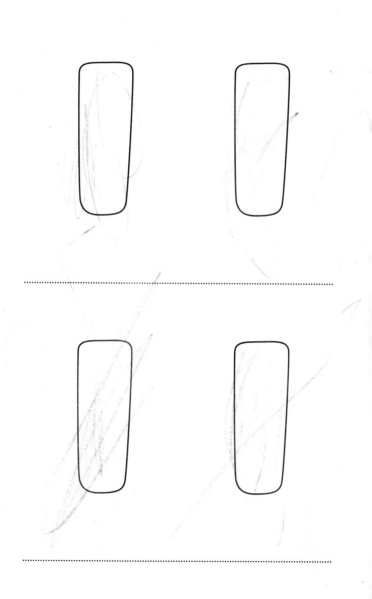

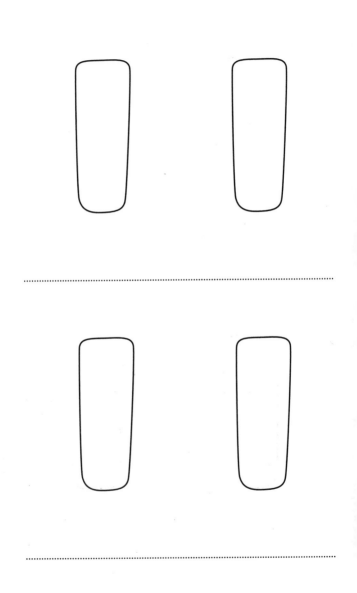

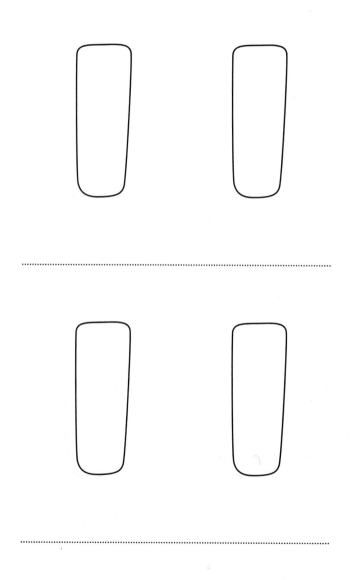

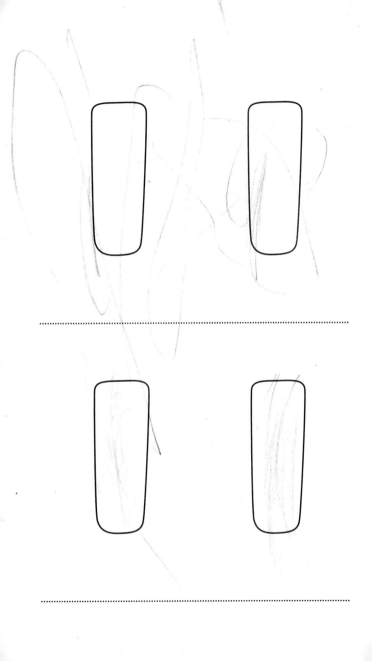

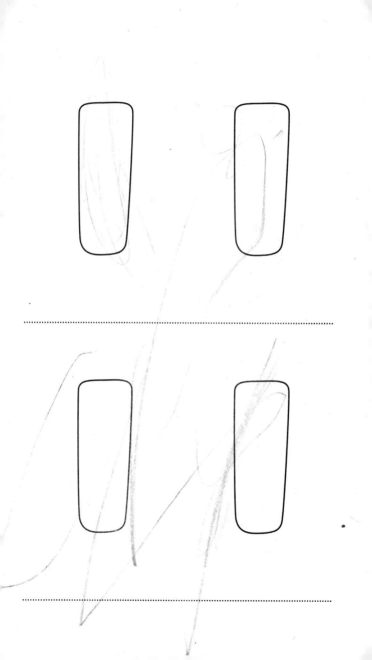

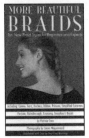
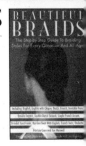
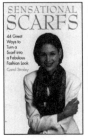
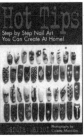